WALL PILATES WORKOUT

Maria Fraley

Keep in mind: Always seek advice from a healthcare expert before embarking on any new fitness regimen. You must assess your own medical and physical state and independently decide whether to engage in, apply, or modify any of the information or content within this publication. Any fitness regimen can potentially lead to injuries. By voluntarily participating in any of the exercises shown in this publication, you accept the risk of any potential injury.

TABLE OF CONTENTS

INTRODUCTION

Welcome, dear reader, to the captivating world of Wall Pilates. On this transformative journey with you, I am committed to offering an experience that fosters physical health and mental strength. The core aim of this book is to equip you with insights, guide you on your fitness path, and instill an enduring drive for holistic health and well-being.

Wall Pilates, an underappreciated yet significantly potent exercise method, stands as a hidden treasure in the world of fitness. Its essence lies in its simplicity and versatility, transforming a mere wall into a tool for strength, flexibility, and overall health. Visualize enjoying the perks of a well-rounded fitness routine from the coziness of your own home, using nothing more than a humble wall. Fascinating, right?

Within this book, i will reveal this mighty discipline in its full grandeur. Whether you are an ardent fitness enthusiast or someone just starting on your wellness journey, Wall Pilates holds the promise of a healthier, stronger you. It is my aim to make this art accessible and understandable, offering you the tools to build a healthier and more balanced life.

Each chapter of this book has been meticulously crafted to unfold the secrets of Wall Pilates gradually. From understanding the principles that underpin this discipline to detailed exercise descriptions to curated workout plans designed to suit diverse needs – every aspect has been covered comprehensively.

However, as we advance, bear in mind that the true charm of Wall Pilates resides not only in the physical movements but in the deep bond it cultivates among body, mind, and spirit. I welcome you to plunge into this journey and witness the transformation personally.

But as we embark on this journey together, I wish to acknowledge that your feedback holds great importance. It would be my absolute pleasure to hear about your Wall Pilates journey. The refinement of this work heavily relies on your insights, recommendations, and constructive feedback. Upon completion of this book, I would greatly appreciate your reflections and critique. Your backing would be instrumental in disseminating this work. This entire book is evidence of my unwavering commitment and zeal. I hope you find this article entertaining and, more importantly, helpful in your pursuit of a happier and healthier lifestyle.

UNDERSTANDING WALL PILATES

Have you ever aspired to have a fitness regimen that not only assists in attaining your objectives but also caters to your craving for variety and originality? If your answer is yes, then enter the world of Wall Pilates, an intriguing and challenging variant of traditional Pilates that infuses an inventive twist into your fitness voyage. And it's just the beginning. As we journey together through this book, there are countless unique facets of Wall Pilates that you'll discover - secrets that will transform your approach to fitness.

Wall Pilates is essentially a fusion of Pilates principles with the added challenge and support of a vertical plane, which is a wall. This type of workout offers an expansive range of exercises that enhances your body's strength, balance, and flexibility, while also providing you with the opportunity to get creative with your workouts.

Benefits of Wall Pilate

1. Improving Balance and Flexibility
One of the key benefits of Wall Pilates is its potential for improving balance and flexibility. The exercises emphasize measured movements, and by using the wall as a support and resistance system, you oppose gravity in a manner that remarkably enhances your balance. As you advance, your body adapts, achieving enhanced flexibility that allows for smoother and more fluid movements.

2. Pain Relief
The beauty of Wall Pilates is its ability to offer a diverse array of health and fitness benefits, many of which extend beyond what traditional Pilates or even yoga provides. Just to name a few, Wall Pilates helps to alleviate low back pain, soothe neck muscle strain, manage conditions like cox-arthrosis, osteoporosis, and more. It serves as a robust tool for maintaining pelvic and back mobility, particularly in individuals suffering from poor posture.

3. Weight loss and Strength Gain
For those interested in weight loss and strength gain, Wall Pilates delivers. The unexpected caloric burn during these exercises often delights many. Besides assisting in weight reduction, these workouts contribute to enhancing muscle strength and definition. After all, in Wall Pilates, you are constantly working against the force of gravity and your body weight, leading to increased muscle definition and strength.

4. Recovery from Trauma or Accidents
Moreover, Wall Pilates can be a powerful aid in recovery from trauma or accidents. Its gentler, controlled movements offer a safe way to start rebuilding strength and mobility without putting excessive strain on the body.

5. Mental Health Benefits

Just like classic Pilates and yoga, Wall Pilates also emphasizes the mind-body connection. This mindful way of exercising can help reduce stress, promote relaxation, and improve overall mental well-being.

6. Increased Body Awareness

Wall Pilates exercises require precision and control, which improves proprioception - our sense of body position. This heightened body awareness can lead to improved movement efficiency not just in workouts but in daily life as well.

Wall Pilates offers a holistic approach to health and well-being. It's more than just an exercise routine; it's a method of boosting physical health and nurturing a conscious interaction with your body. With consistent practice, you'll harvest the multitude of benefits this adaptable and efficient workout system presents.

Wall Pilates, Yoga, and Classic Pilates – How do they compare?

The brilliance of Wall Pilates is its inclusivity, making it appropriate for a wide array of individuals. Regardless of your age, fitness level, or health status, there's a spot for you in the world of Wall Pilates.

The following is how diverse groups can take advantage of this distinctive exercise regimen:

• **Fitness Beginners**

For those who are new to exercise, Wall Pilates offers a safe and supportive way to get started. The wall serves as a prop, offering stability and support that can help build confidence and strength. The variety of exercises also keeps workouts interesting, which can motivate newcomers to stick with their fitness journey.

• **Intermediate to Advanced Exercisers**

For those with a certain level of fitness, Wall Pilates serves as an excellent tool for diversification and further development. The unique challenges offered by the vertical plane can help to improve core strength, flexibility, and balance, pushing fitness boundaries and driving progress.

• **Older Adults**

Wall Pilates is a gentle yet effective workout choice for older adults. The focus on core strength, flexibility, and balance is particularly beneficial for this demographic, as these aspects are vital to maintaining independence and preventing falls. Furthermore, the wall provides a level of support and stability that can boost confidence and make exercise more accessible.

• **Individuals with Special Considerations**

Wall Pilates can be a gentle and controlled way for those recovering from an injury or managing chronic health conditions to regain strength and mobility. The opportunity to use the wall for support and balance makes it a safe choice. However, it is essential for these individuals to obtain guidance from health practitioners or trained professionals to ensure that the exercises are suitable and advantageous for their unique situations.

• Expectant and Postnatal Women

With the proper modifications and precautions, Wall Pilates can be a great way to maintain fitness during and after pregnancy. The focus on core and pelvic floor strength can be particularly beneficial. As always, consulting with a healthcare provider before starting or continuing any exercise program during this time is essential.

Whether you want to start your fitness journey, diversify your workouts, or find a gentle way to stay active, Wall Pilates has something to offer.

Muscles Targeted in Wall Pilates

Wall Pilates is a comprehensive workout method that targets multiple muscle groups across the body.

The following are the specific muscles that Wall Pilates works:

• Core Muscles

Like traditional Pilates, Wall Pilates places a significant focus on core strength. This includes the "six-pack" muscle (rectus abdominis), the obliques (muscles on the sides of your abdomen), and the transverse abdominis (deep muscles that wrap around your spine and flanks). These muscles are engaged during the exercise to offer body stability and spinal support.

• Back Muscles

Wall Pilates exercises are designed to strengthen the entire back. This includes the large muscles in the lower back (erector spinae), the muscles between the shoulder blades (rhomboids), and the muscles along the spine (multifidi). Strengthening these muscles supports proper posture and spinal health.

• Hip and Glute Muscles

Multiple Wall Pilates movements target the muscles in the hip and gluteal area, such as the gluteus maximus, gluteus medius, and gluteus minimus. These movements play a role in contouring and strengthening these muscles, simultaneously improving balance and steadiness.

• Thigh and Leg Muscles

Wall Pilates is effective in targeting both the anterior (frontal) and posterior (rear) muscles of the thighs and legs, incorporating the quadriceps, hamstrings, and calf muscles. The wall offers resistance for these exercises, assisting in building strength and stamina.

• Shoulder and Arm Muscles

While not as intensely focused on as the core, back, and lower body, Wall Pilates does engage the upper body muscles. This refers to the deltoids in the shoulders, the biceps and triceps in the arms, and the pectorals in the chest.

• Pelvic Floor Muscles

Wall Pilates also stimulates the pelvic floor muscles, a group of muscles offering support to your pelvic organs. Strengthening these muscles can alleviate or improve conditions like incontinence and pelvic organ descent.

The holistic nature of Wall Pilates means that it doesn't isolate one muscle group while ignoring the others. Instead, it works to strengthen the body as a whole, which means that it is an effective workout for overall body conditioning and health improvement.

Calorie Burn Information

A common question about any fitness regimen is its calorie-burning potential. Understanding how many calories a particular exercise or routine burns can be a crucial factor for individuals aiming for weight loss or maintaining a healthy weight.

While the precise number of calories burned during a Wall Pilates session can differ significantly depending on various factors, including:
- **Weight:** Heavier individuals burn more calories as it requires more energy (calories) to move a larger body.
- **Age:** Generally, with aging comes a decrease in metabolic rate, resulting in fewer calories burnt during physical activities.
- **Gender:** Males usually expend more calories than females during identical activities, mainly because of their greater muscle mass.
- **Intensity:** The tougher your workout is, the more calories you expend. This is relevant both to the hardness level of the exercises and the speed at which you execute them.

On average, a moderate-intensity Wall Pilates workout of one hour can burn anywhere between 200 to 400 calories. This estimate is quite broad and should be used as a rough guide rather than an exact figure. For reference, this calorie burn range is akin to a brisk walk or a slow bicycle ride. It's less than what you'd burn during a vigorous activity like running, but it can be more than traditional mat Pilates or gentle yoga, especially considering the added resistance and challenge provided by the wall.

It's important to remember that the total calories burned are only part of the equation when it comes to weight loss or maintenance. The diet also plays a crucial role. To lose weight, the calories burned must exceed the calories consumed, creating a calorie deficit.

Importance of Nutrition

While physical exercise is a critical component of a healthy lifestyle, it's just one part of the equation. Nutrition holds equal, if not more excellent, significance. Without appropriate nutrition, your body might lack the energy it needs to function optimally, and you may not achieve the results you anticipate. Let's delve into why nutrition is so important when following a Wall Pilates regimen, or any fitness program for that matter.

• Fuel for Your Workouts

Your body draws energy from the food you eat to perform its functions. A healthy diet makes sure your body has the resources it needs to power your Wall Pilates routines. This includes carbohydrates for quick energy, proteins for muscle repair and recovery, and fats for sustained energy.

• Optimizing Recovery

After a strenuous Wall Pilates session, your muscles need nutrients to recover and grow stronger. Top-tier proteins and complex carbohydrates are instrumental in this process.

• Supporting Weight Management

If weight reduction is your objective, pairing Wall Pilates with a calorie-restricted diet can be effective. Creating a calorie deficit—expending more calories than consumed—is a crucial aspect of weight loss. At the same time, a balanced diet guarantees you're receiving the broad array of nutrients essential for health and wellness.

• Enhancing Overall Health

Good nutrition is vital for more than just physical fitness. It supports all physical processes, helps in warding off diseases, and affects mood and mental health. Your overall health and wellness will improve a lot if you eat a lot of fruits, lean proteins, whole grains, vegetables, and healthy fats.

• Strengthening Bones

Wall Pilates is celebrated for its focus on enhancing balance and flexibility, which are crucial for maintaining bone health. A nutrient-rich diet, especially one abundant in calcium and vitamin D, is vital for keeping bones robust and healthy.

• Promoting Gut Health

A diet rich in fiber can foster a healthy gut. A sturdy gut can aid in digestion, enhance nutrient uptake, and strengthen the immune system.

It's apparent that diet and exercise are two intertwined aspects in the promotion of health, fitness, and well-being. Adhering to a balanced diet alongside your Wall Pilates regimen can aid in attaining your fitness objectives and augmenting your overall health.

As we close this chapter, here's a teaser for the next one: "How does something as simple as breathing influence our Wall Pilates practice? What's the connection between slow, deliberate movements and our mind-body harmony?" Intrigued? Chapter 2 has all the answers. Let's take this fascinating journey together.

BREATHWORK AND SLOW MOVEMENTS IN WALL PILATES

Welcome to the next phase of your Wall Pilates journey! As we delve deeper into the multifaceted world of Wall Pilates, we're bound to uncover numerous revelations, the significance of breathing and slow movements being among the first. In this chapter, we'll explore how these two seemingly simple elements lay the foundation of Wall Pilates and elevate the practice to a holistic exercise method. Ready to unlock the mysteries? Let's get started!

The Life Force: Breathwork in Wall Pilates

Breathing – it's an essential life process, something we do without conscious thought. Yet, when it comes to Wall Pilates, conscious breathing takes center stage. Breathing is not merely a passive player; it is a critical component that can enhance or even transform your Wall Pilates experience.

When practicing Pilates, there is a specific breathing technique referred to as "lateral" or "thoracic" breathing. This approach emphasizes the intake of deep breaths through the nasal passages. The method involves expanding the chest not only in the anterior direction but also towards the sides and the posterior region. When exhaling, typically through the mouth, you engage in a deliberate, robust process, pulling your abdominal muscles inward and upward, envisioning your navel moving towards your spine. This engagement of the abdominal muscles on exhalation forms the basis of the core work in Pilates.

The following is the importance of breathing in Wall Pilates:
1. Enhances Core Engagement
The Pilates breathing technique encourages active engagement of the core. When you exhale forcefully and pull your abdominals in and up, you're essentially activating and training your deep core muscles, including the transverse abdominis and pelvic floor muscles. This not only strengthens your core but also supports spine stability and promotes better body mechanics.

2. Improves Oxygenation
Conscious, deep breathing improves the oxygen supply to your muscles and brain. This enhances the efficiency of your workout and promotes better concentration, allowing you to perform exercises with greater precision and control.

3. Facilitates Movement
In Wall Pilates, breath is synchronized with Movement. Typically, you exhale on the effort or exertion part of an exercise and inhale on the release. This rhythmic coordination helps facilitate Movement, making it more fluid and efficient.

4. Promotes Relaxation
Concentrating on your breath can induce a sense of calm in your mind. It helps you remain in the moment, alleviates stress, and encourages a feeling of relaxation. This is

particularly beneficial in today's fast-paced, often stressful world, making Wall Pilates not just a physical exercise but also a form of moving meditation.

5. Aids in Body Awareness
Paying attention to your breath can heighten body awareness. It promotes mindfulness and helps you tune into your body's needs and responses, fostering a deeper mind-body connection.

6. Supports Proper Posture
Active engagement of the core through Pilates breathing supports better posture. This helps to preserve the natural arch of the spine, reducing the chances of back ailments and other musculoskeletal disorders.

7. Detoxification
A forceful exhale assists in ejecting carbon dioxide, a byproduct of metabolism, from your body. This "internal cleansing" aspect of Pilates breathing promotes better overall health.

Understanding and practicing the Pilates breathing technique can profoundly impact your Wall Pilates experience. It helps transform your workouts from mere physical exertion to a holistic mind-body practice that enhances strength, flexibility, and overall well-being.

Emphasizing Slow Movements

Wall Pilates distinguishes itself by concentrating on slow, measured movements in a society fixated on high-intensity, fast-moving workouts. This method is not about simplifying the workout; it's about making it more mindful and efficient.

Here's why emphasizing slow movements is so crucial in Wall Pilates:
1. Promotes Precision
Slow movements allow for more precise execution. Pilates doesn't focus on the number of repetitions; it concentrates on their quality. Slowing down provides the time and space to ensure accurate alignment and form, making the exercise more efficient and reducing injury risk.

2. Enhances Mind-Body Connection
Slow movements require more conscious control, enhancing the mind-body connection. This mindfulness element makes Pilates not just a physical workout but also a form of moving meditation that can boost mental well-being.

3. Increases Muscle Activation
Slow, controlled movements typically involve more muscle tension over a more extended period. This can increase muscle activation, especially in stabilizing muscles, making the exercise more challenging and improving strength gains.

4. Fosters Core Strength

In Pilates, slow movements, combined with the conscious engagement of the core (as emphasized by the unique Pilates breathing technique), foster deep core strength. This is essential for improving posture, balance, and overall functional fitness.

5. Improves Balance
Slow movements require and improve balance. By moving slowly, you challenge your body's proprioception (the sense of self-movement and body position), helping to improve stability and coordination.

6. Enhances Flexibility
When you perform movements slowly, you allow your muscles time to lengthen and stretch. This can enhance flexibility over time.

7. Teaches Patience
In a broader sense, the emphasis on slow movements in Wall Pilates also teaches patience and the ability to be fully present in the moment. This can have benefits beyond your physical fitness, positively impacting your overall mental and emotional well-being.

8. Boosts Metabolic Efficiency
Slow and controlled movements, especially when they involve maintaining a position or muscle contraction, can boost metabolic efficiency by improving muscular endurance and promoting lean muscle mass.

As you can see, slowing down in Wall Pilates is about more than just making the workout easier. Instead, it's a deliberate approach that applies the principles of biomechanics, mindfulness, and physiology to increase the efficacy of your workout.

Connection Between Body and Soul

The unique charm of Wall Pilates doesn't just lie in its physical advantages but also in the deep connection it nurtures between the body and spirit. This aspect originates in the comprehensive philosophy of Joseph Pilates, who envisioned his method as a means of synchronizing the body, mind, and spirit.

So, how does Wall Pilates establish this connection? Let's explore:
• **Promoting Mindfulness**
Wall Pilates, focusing on slow, controlled movements and conscious breathing, naturally cultivates mindfulness. Every Movement demands your full attention, grounding you in the present moment. This type of focused presence is a form of mindfulness practice associated with stress reduction, improved mental focus, and enhanced emotional well-being.

• **Enhancing Body Awareness**
The precision required in Wall Pilates significantly improves your proprioception or your body's sense of where it is in space. This increased body consciousness can lead to a

deeper understanding of your physical self, intensifying the connection between your body and mindful awareness.

• Emotional Release
Physical Movement can be a powerful tool for emotional release. As you engage with your body in Wall Pilates, you might experience various emotional states. Embracing these emotions rather than suppressing them can lead to better emotional regulation and a deeper connection with your inner self.

• Harmonizing Energy
Pilates is often thought of as a moving meditation. By focusing on the breath, one can improve physical function and balance the body's energy. This equilibrium can foster a feeling of peace and tranquillity, connecting the physical body and the spirit.

• Nurturing Self-Love
Wall Pilates cultivates an attitude of patience, kindness, and respect toward your body, irrespective of your abilities or fitness level. This practice of self-appreciation and acceptance can lead to an improved body image and a stronger connection with your inner self.

• Building Resilience
The physical challenge of Wall Pilates can also build mental resilience. Each time you overcome a challenging posture or hold a difficult pose for a few breaths longer, you're training your mind to cope with discomfort, fostering mental strength and resilience.

The connection between body and soul in Wall Pilates goes beyond simple fitness. It's about holistic well-being, embodying a philosophy that acknowledges the interrelation of physical, mental, and emotional health.

In Wall Pilates, the breath becomes our guide, and slow movements become our dance. Collectively, they establish the cadence of our practice, setting the pace for a workout that transforms us, not just physically but also mentally and emotionally.

In our subsequent chapter, we'll transition our focus towards the precautions necessary while practicing Wall Pilates. From maintaining proper alignment to ensuring a high level of concentration, we'll uncover how to make your Wall Pilates experience not just effective but also safe.

SAFETY PRECAUTIONS IN WALL PILATES

The beauty and efficiency of Wall Pilates lie in its simplicity. However, like any other physical activity, safety precautions are integral to its practice. This chapter will lead you on a journey of understanding the safety precautions in Wall Pilates, arming you with the necessary knowledge to embark on your Wall Pilates journey securely and confidently.

Precautions to Avoid Injury

The philosophy of Wall Pilates, much like any other exercise routine, centers on the idea of nurturing one's body rather than causing it harm. Consequently, implementing precautionary steps to avert injuries is a vital aspect of the practice.

Take into account the following:
• **Ensure a Safe Environment**
Your exercise area should be devoid of any potential hazards. Ensure there is ample space for you to move freely without colliding with furniture or other obstacles. The wall you're utilizing for the exercise should be stable and even. Remove any hanging pictures or other decorations that could potentially fall or be knocked down during your workout.

• **Appropriate Warm-up and Cool-down**
Inadequate warm-up before starting and cool-down after completing the workout is a frequent cause of injury during physical activities. A warm-up enhances your body temperature and blood circulation, preparing your muscles and joints for the forthcoming activity. Conversely, a cool-down aids your body in returning to its resting state, reducing the risk of muscle rigidity or a sudden drop in blood pressure.

• **Listen to Your Body**
Each person is unique concerning flexibility, strength, and endurance. It's imperative to listen to your body and respect its limitations. Should you feel any pain during a workout, halt immediately. Discomfort is your body's way of signaling that something isn't right. Also, advance at your own speed, intensifying the exercises gradually.

• **Use the Correct Equipment**
If your routine includes any equipment, such as resistance bands or small balls, make sure they're in good condition and safe to use. Using faulty equipment can lead to unexpected accidents and injuries.

• **Stay Hydrated**
Maintaining proper fluid balance is essential for your well-being, as inadequate hydration may result in different bodily concerns, such as muscle discomfort and a feeling of dizziness. To restore the lost fluids due to sweating, it is vital to ensure sufficient water intake before, during, and after your exercise routine.

• **Healthy Nutrition**

Proper nutrition is crucial for physical activities like Pilates. Your body requires sufficient nutrients for muscle building and repair, bone health maintenance, and providing energy for your workouts. A balanced diet can help prevent injuries linked to nutrient deficiencies and boost your overall performance.

Importance of Correct Form and Alignment

Just like a beautiful building needs a solid foundation and structure, a good Pilates practice is grounded in the principles of correct form and alignment. This crucial aspect of Wall Pilates not only optimizes your workouts but also prevents injuries and enhances overall body health.

Here's the importance of correct form and alignment:
• Promotes Efficiency

Proper form and alignment ensure that the right muscles are working during each exercise. This maximizes the effectiveness of each Movement, making your workout more efficient and results-driven. With correct form, you may fully activate the intended muscles, leading to less effective workouts.

• Prevents Injuries

Incorrect form and alignment can place undue strain on the wrong muscles or joints, leading to potential injuries. For example, if your alignment is off during a leg lift, you might strain your back instead of working your core. Maintaining correct form reduces the risk of such mishaps.

• Improves Posture

Regular Wall Pilates workouts with the correct form can significantly enhance your posture. This can alleviate ailments like back pain and neck tension that often result from poor posture. Moreover, good posture can boost your confidence and improve your overall appearance.

• Enhances Body Awareness

Focusing on form and alignment necessitates mindfulness and body awareness. This can enhance your proprioception - your sense of your body's position and Movement in space, which is vital for coordination and movement efficiency.

• Facilitates Balance and Symmetry

Correct alignment ensures equilibrium between the left and right sides of the body and between different muscle groups. This aids in avoiding muscular imbalances, which could lead to discomfort and injury over time.

• Accelerates Progress

With appropriate form and alignment, you'll execute each exercise as it's intended, which will fast-track your progress toward your fitness objectives.

To ensure accurate form and alignment, consider collaborating with a certified Pilates instructor who can offer personalized advice. Remember it's not about how many exercises you complete but how well you execute them. After all, in Wall Pilates - and in any form of exercise - quality always trumps quantity!

Maintaining Concentration During Workouts

In the rapid-paced world, we inhabit, maintaining focus, particularly during physical activities like Pilates, can appear challenging. Nonetheless, it is vital for maximizing benefits and reducing the risk of injury.

The following are the reasons why concentration is vital and how to maintain it during your Wall Pilates workouts:

• Safety

Properly executed Pilates movements require a high degree of attention to detail. By ensuring that you maintain perfect form and alignment throughout your workout, being focused lowers your chance of injury. This is especially important in Wall Pilates, where the wall serves as a point of contact, support, and resistance.

• Effectiveness

Concentration is critical for the mind-muscle connection, where you actively think about the muscle you're engaging in during an exercise. This connection can increase the effectiveness of your workouts by ensuring that the correct muscle groups are targeted.

• Mind-Body Connection

Pilates is a mind-body exercise. By focusing on each Movement, you become more in tune with your body and its capabilities. This can lead to enhanced proprioception and body awareness, fostering balance, coordination, and flexibility.

• Stress Reduction

Focusing on your movements allows you to be in the present moment, which can help clear your mind from daily stressors and promote mental well-being. The mind-body connection in Pilates can be a form of meditation in motion.

So how can you improve your concentration during workouts?

1. **Set Clear Intentions:** Before you start, understand what you want to achieve in the workout. Having a clear goal will help to maintain your focus and purpose.
2. **Limit Distractions:** Try to set up your workout space in a quiet, calm area. This could involve turning off notifications on your phone or informing your family or roommates about your workout time.
3. **Focus on Breathing:** Your breath can be a powerful tool to center your attention. In Pilates, each Movement is coordinated with the breath, which helps keep you engaged.
4. **Quality over Quantity:** Rather than rushing through the exercises, take your time. This helps keep your focus on the form and execution of each Movement.

By cultivating concentration during your Wall Pilates sessions, you'll be able to delve deeper into your practice and fully reap the physical and mental benefits that Pilates has to offer.

Safety precautions are the foundation of any beneficial Wall Pilates practice. They help create a balanced, sustainable, and effective workout experience. Remember, Pilates isn't about pushing your body to its limits; it's about finding harmony between body and soul while promoting health and well-being.

EQUIPMENT FOR WALL PILATES

As we delve deeper into the intriguing world of Wall Pilates, it's evident that the equipment utilized plays a significant role in enhancing our practice and strengthening our bond with this exercise form. This chapter will shed light on the various types of equipment commonly employed in Wall Pilates and guide you to select the suitable ones for your needs.

Understanding Wall Pilates Equipment

Wall Pilates often requires minimal equipment, and this simplicity is part of its charm. However, some tools can make the practice more efficient, safer, and customizable to your needs.

Here are some of the most commonly used equipment in Wall Pilates:

1. Wall Unit

The Wall Unit is the fundamental piece of equipment in Wall Pilates. It consists of a wall-mounted structure that has a mat and several spring attachments. Springs are a critical component of the Wall Unit, as they offer adjustable resistance that can be tailored to match your strength and desired workout intensity. They assist in targeting different muscle groups and permit a wide array of exercises, contributing to the development of strength, flexibility, and balance.

2. Pilates Mat

The mat used in Wall Pilates is different from your typical yoga mat. A Pilates mat is thicker, providing more cushioning to support your spine, joints, and bones during exercises. This extra padding is especially essential during exercises where you are lying down, kneeling, or sitting.

3. Pilates Ring

Also known as the Magic Circle, the Pilates Ring is a flexible ring with pads on the sides. It's used in various exercises to provide added resistance and assist with alignment. The ring can be squeezed between the hands, the thighs, or the ankles to engage and strengthen specific muscle groups.

4. Resistance Bands

Resistance bands are elastic bands that can be used to modify the intensity of your workouts. They can be used in a similar way to the springs on the Wall Unit, offering resistance that can be adjusted according to your fitness level. They are particularly beneficial for those who need a lower-impact workout or are rehabilitating from an injury.

5. Stability Ball

This large inflatable ball is used to challenge balance and engage the core muscles during Wall Pilates workouts. By performing exercises on the unstable surface of the ball, you force your body to confront multiple muscle groups at once, leading to improved strength and stability.

Understanding each piece of Wall Pilates equipment and its uses can enhance your workouts and ensure you are performing exercises safely and effectively.

Choosing the Right Equipment

Making the right equipment selection is a crucial step in your Wall Pilates journey.

Here's all you need to consider:
• Understanding Your Needs
The initial step in selecting the appropriate equipment is understanding your needs and objectives. Are your goals centered around enhancing strength, boosting flexibility, recovering from an injury, or blending these? Once your fitness goals are clear, you can begin to discern which equipment pieces will aid you most effectively in reaching these goals. For instance, if flexibility is your primary goal, you might focus on equipment like resistance bands and the Pilates Ring.

• Consult a Professional
If you're a newcomer to Wall Pilates, seeking advice from a Pilates instructor or a fitness professional is recommended. They can offer expert insights on the kind of equipment that would be most beneficial for you, considering your fitness level, objectives, and any physical restrictions or health concerns you might possess.

• Quality Over Quantity
When choosing equipment, prioritize quality over quantity. While high-quality, durable equipment might come with a higher price tag, its longevity and contribution to a safer, more efficient workout make it a worthwhile investment. Inexpensive, low-quality equipment can break easily, posing potential injury risks. It's prudent to check reviews and conduct some research before deciding on a purchase.

• Comfort and Fit
Make sure the equipment is comfortable and fits well with your body. This is especially crucial for equipment like the Wall Unit, which should be adjusted to your height and flexibility level. If buying a Pilates mat, ensure it provides enough cushioning to support your body during exercises.

• Space Considerations
Be mindful of the space where you will be conducting your workouts. Some Wall Pilates equipment, like the Wall Unit, requires significant space for installation and use. Measure your space beforehand to ensure the equipment will fit appropriately.

With the correct equipment, you can maximize your workout's effectiveness and enjoy your Pilates journey fully.

WARM-UP EXERCISES

Wall Mountain Climbers

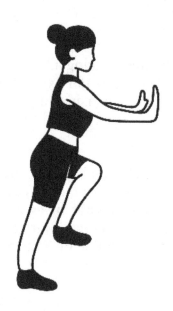

1. Start in a high plank position with your hands flat on the wall, your wrists under your shoulders, and your feet hip-width apart.
2. Draw your right knee towards your chest, striving for maximum proximity. Alternate legs, extending one knee outward while pulling the other knee inward.
3. Run your knees in and out as fast as you can, keeping your core engaged.
4. Repeat this Movement 20 times (10 for each leg).

Wall Lunges

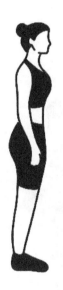 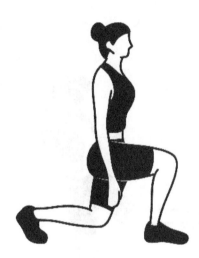

1. Stand a few feet away from the wall with your back facing it.
2. Take a step forward with your right foot.
3. Gradually flex your knees to descend into a lunge, ensuring that your right knee remains directly aligned with your right ankle while the left knee maintains a downward orientation towards the floor.
4. Push back up to standing and switch legs.
5. Perform this motion in a repetitive manner, executing it a total of 10 times for each leg.

Wall Leg Swings

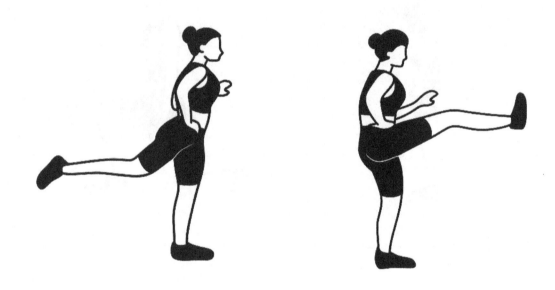

1. Stand facing the wall, about arm's length away.
2. Place your hands on the wall for support and shift your weight onto one foot.
3. Swing your other leg forward and backward in a controlled motion.
4. Repeat 10-12 times on each leg.

Wall Single-Leg Lifts

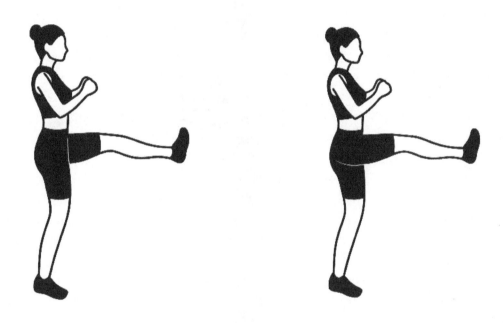

1. Stand a few feet away from the wall, facing it.
2. Extend your right leg out in front of you while keeping your balance on your left foot.
3. Lift your right leg as high as possible, then lower it back down.
4. Repeat this Movement 10-12 times, then switch to the left leg.

Wall Calf Raises

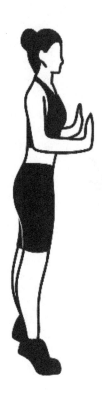

1. Stand facing the wall with your hands at chest level against the wall for balance.
2. Lift your heels off the ground as high as possible, balancing on the balls of your feet.
3. Lower your heels back down to the ground.
4. Repeat this Movement 15-20 times.

STRENGTH TRAINING EXERCISE

Downward Dog

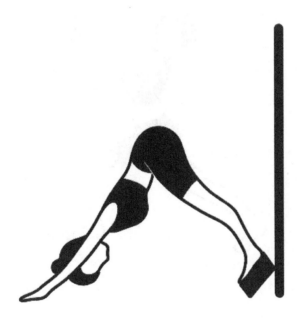

1. Start in the Downward Facing Dog position with your hands on the floor and your feet against the wall.
2. Try to get your heels as close to the wall as possible, and push your chest towards your knees to deepen the stretch.
3. Engage your core and keep your gaze towards your feet.
4. Hold this position for 30-60 seconds.

High Lunge Pose

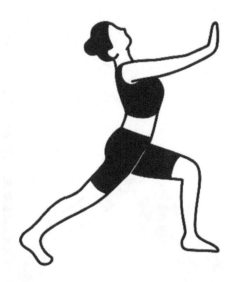

1. Stand facing the wall with your arms reaching upwards and your palms against the wall.
2. Take a big step back with your right foot and lower your right knee until it's just above the ground. Make sure your left knee is aligned with your left ankle and not passing your toes. Engage your core and press your right heel towards the back of the room.
3. Hold this pose for 30-60 seconds, then switch legs.

Wall Squats

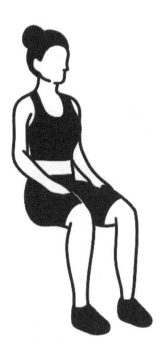

1. Start by standing with your back against the wall. Position your feet about shoulder-width apart, roughly two feet away from the wall.
2. Keep your arms either stretched out in front of you or resting on your hips, whichever you find more comfortable.
3. Slowly bend your knees, sliding your back down the wall until your thighs are parallel to the ground, ensuring that your knees are directly above your ankles. Your body should resemble sitting on an invisible chair. During this exercise, avoid arching your back or tilting your pelvis too far forward or backward.
4. Hold this position for a moment, keeping your core engaged. Ensure not to let your knees cave inward; they should stay directly over your ankles.
5. Slowly stand back up by straightening your knees and pushing your body upwards.
6. Repeat this Movement 10-12 times.

Wall Push-Ups

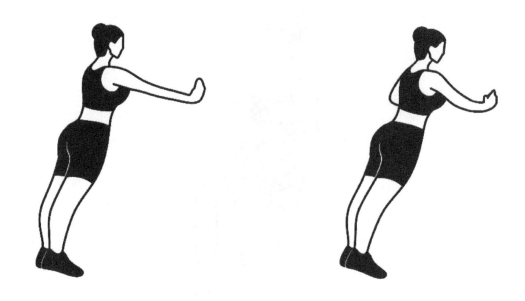

1. Stand a couple of feet away from the wall, facing it. The exact distance will depend on your height, but you should be far enough to fully extend your arms and place your palms flat against the wall without leaning into it.
2. Keep your feet shoulder-width apart, firmly planted on the ground.
3. Place your hands on the wall, shoulder-width apart. Your hands should be at chest level.
4. Slowly bend your elbows, bringing your chest closer to the wall. Keep your body straight from your head to your heels, avoiding sagging hips or a hyperextended neck.
5. Once your elbows are at about a 90-degree angle or slightly less, pause for a moment and avoid locking your elbows or pushing too far, which could lead to strain.
6. Push your body back to the starting position, extending your arms fully without locking the elbows.
7. Repeat this Movement 10-12 times.

Wall Plank

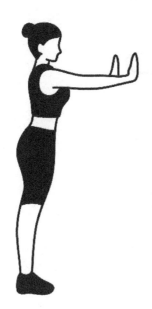 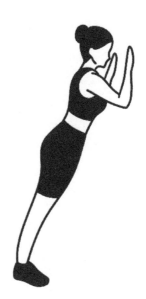

1. Stand facing the wall, a little farther than arm's length away.
2. Lean forward, placing your palms on the wall.
3. Walk your feet backward until your body is at an incline, parallel to the ground.
4. Hold this position for 30-60 seconds.

Wall Tuck and Extend

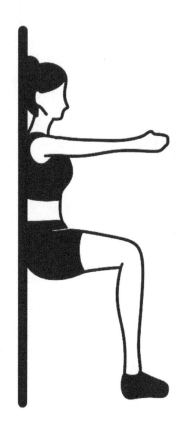

1. Stand facing away from the wall with your feet shoulder-width apart.
2. Extend your arms forward, bend your knees, and lean your hips into the wall, coming into a squat position.
3. Extend your legs and stand tall, reaching your arms up over your head.
4. Repeat this Movement 10-12 times.

Wall Side Plank

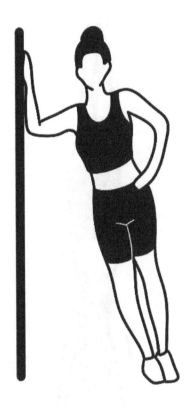

1. Stand sideways to the wall, feet together.
2. Lean onto your closest hand, keeping it directly under your shoulder.
3. Stack your feet and lift your hips, creating a straight line from your head to your feet.
4. Hold this position for 30-60 seconds, then switch sides.

Wall Handstand

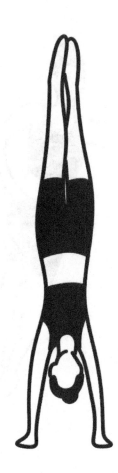

1. Stand facing away from the wall.
2. Place your hands on the floor a few feet away from the wall and kick your feet up onto the wall.
3. Maintain a straight alignment of your body while distributing the weight evenly between both hands.
4. Hold this position for as long as comfortable, then carefully descend.

Wall Sit with Mini Fitness Ball

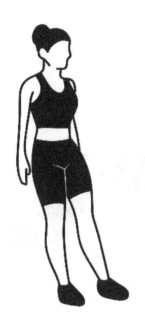 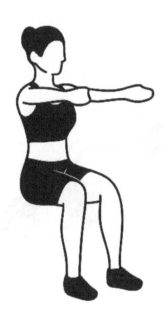

1. Position a mini fitness ball between your lower back and the wall.
2. Stand with your feet shoulder-width apart.
3. Gently slide your back against the wall, gradually lowering your knees until they form a 90-degree angle, allowing for a slight descent of the ball during the Movement.
4. Ensure your thighs are parallel to the ground and your knees are directly above your ankles.
5. Maintain this stance for 30 to 60 seconds, focusing on engaging your core muscles to stabilize the ball.
6. Slowly slide back up the wall to a standing position, letting the ball roll up with your Movement.

Wall Bridge

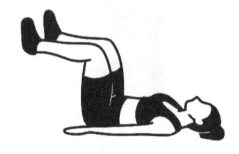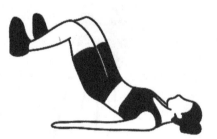

1. Recline on the surface with your feet positioned flush against the wall, your knees bent at a precise 90-degree angle. Activate your core muscles and elevate your hips off the ground, aligning your body into a linear configuration from knees to shoulders. Maintain this pose for a brief duration before gradually descending your hips back to the ground.
2. Repeat this Movement 10-12 times.

Supported Warrior III

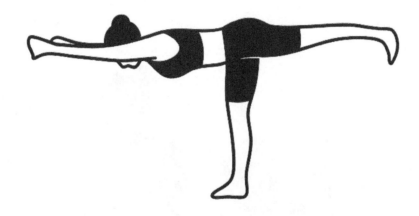

1. Stand facing the wall a few feet away.
2. Extend one leg back, keeping it straight and reaching out with your toes.
3. Lean forward, reaching out with your hands to the wall while maintaining balance on one leg.
4. Hold your body straight from your extended leg to your head.
5. Hold this position for 30-60 seconds, then switch legs.

Wall Sphinx Pose

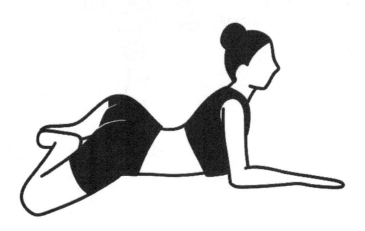

1. Lie on your stomach with your feet against the wall.
2. Prop yourself up on your forearms, aligning your elbows under your shoulders.
3. Exert pressure with your palms and forearms against the floor, raising your chest and generating a mild backbend.
4. Press your feet into the wall to deepen the stretch.
5. Hold this pose for 30-60 seconds.

Four-Limbed Staff Pose Feet Against Wall

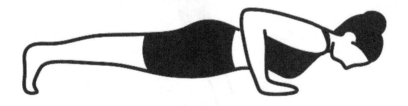

1. Start in a high plank position with your feet against the wall.
2. Gradually descend your body towards the floor by bending your elbows, ensuring they remain in close proximity to your sides.
3. Keep your body in a straight line from your head to your heels.
4. Hold for 10-15 seconds, then push back up to the high plank.

One-Legged Standing Backbend

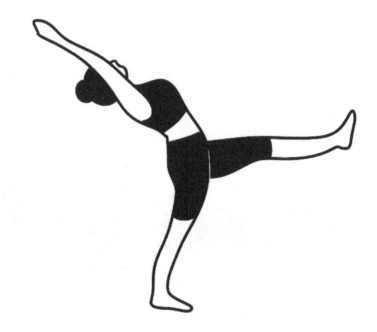

1. Stand a few feet away from the wall with your back to it.
2. Extend your right leg back and place your foot on the wall.
3. Reach your arms back and place your hands on the wall as you bend backward.
4. Hold this pose for 30-60 seconds, then switch sides.

FLEXIBILITY & STRETCHING EXERCISES

Wall Downward Facing Do

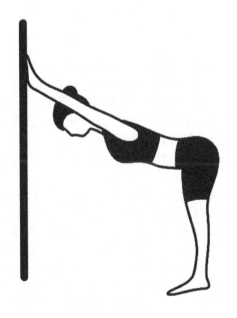

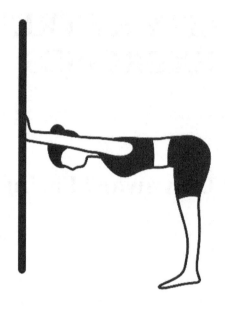

1. Begin by facing the wall. Place your hands on the wall at hip level, about shoulder-width apart. Stand back enough so that your arms are fully extended, but your body is at a slight angle.
2. Position yourself with your feet at a moderate distance from each other and stably grounded, then proceed to move your hips rearward and initiate a forward bend starting from the midsection. Keep your back and arms straight as you do this.
3. Continue the motion of leaning forward and pushing your hips rearward until your body takes on the outline of an upside-down 'V .'Your head should be aligned with your arms, and your gaze should be towards your feet.
4. Make sure to engage your core and maintain a neutral spine. Don't let your lower back sag or your shoulders creep up towards your ears.
5. Hold this position for a few seconds, feeling the stretch in your hamstrings and the strengthening of your arms.
6. Restore yourself to the initial stance by propelling your hips forward and assuming an upright posture.
7. Repeat this Movement 10-12 times.

Wall Slide

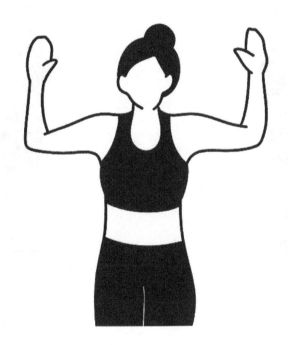

1. Stand with your back against the wall. Your feet should be about shoulder-width apart, roughly two feet away from the wall.
2. Place your arms against the wall in a 'W' shape with your elbows bent at 90 degrees.
3. Slowly slide your arms up the wall into a 'Y' shape, straightening them as you go.
4. Slide them back down to the starting 'W' shape.

Chest Stretch

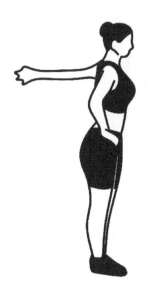 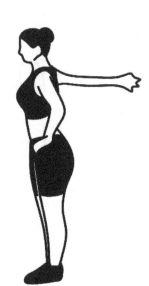

1. Stand sideways to the wall, about arm's length away.
2. Extend the arm closest to the wall straight out and place your palm flat against the wall, fingers pointing straight ahead.
3. Slowly rotate your body away from the wall until you feel a gentle stretch across your chest and front of the shoulder.
4. Maintain this stretched position for a period of 20 to 30 seconds, and subsequently, transition to the opposite side.

Puppy Dog Pose

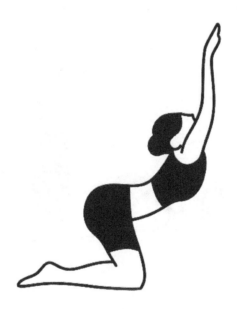

1. Start on all fours, then walk your hands forward until your chest is near the ground.
2. Your hips should be directly above your knees. Extend your arms forward with your palms flat on the wall, spreading your fingers wide.
3. Lower your forehead to the floor, and press your palms to open your chest.
4. Hold this position for 30-60 seconds.

Legs Up The Wall Pose

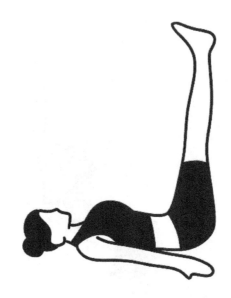

1.   Lie on your back with your legs extended upward against the wall.
2.   Your body should be in an L-shape with your hips close to or touching the wall.
You can place a folded blanket under your lower back for added support.
3.   Hold this position for 3-5 minutes.

Upward Forward Fold

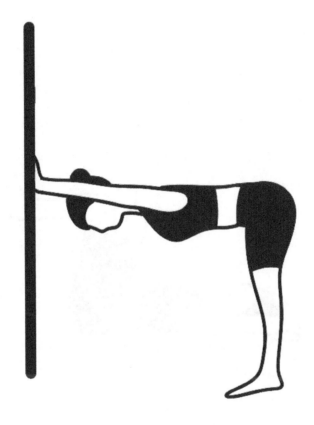

1. Position yourself in a facing stance towards the wall, and proceed to lean forward from your hips while ensuring that your legs remain extended and your hands are flat against the wall at waist height. Your body should form an L shape.
2. Hold this pose for 20-30 seconds.

Sleeping Pigeon Pose

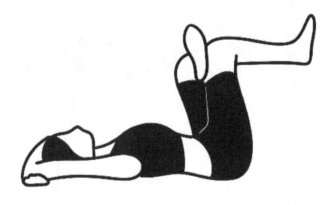

1. Start with your hands and knees on the floor. Bring your right knee forward and place it on the wall, with the right foot pointing to the left side.
2. Extend your left leg straight behind you, ensuring that your hips maintain a squared position and your chest remains lifted. Hold this position for 30-60 seconds, then switch legs.

Eye of The Needle Pose

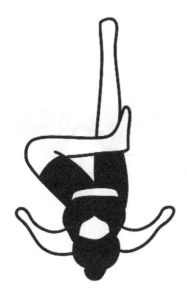

1. Lie on your back with your feet flat on the wall and your knees bent.
2. Cross your right ankle over your left thigh, just above the knee, making a figure-4 shape with your legs.
3. Flex your right foot and press your right knee away from your body.
4. Hold this pose for 30-60 seconds, then switch legs.

Straddle Pose

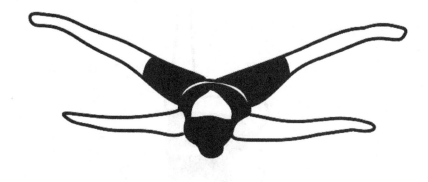

1. Sit down with your legs extended wide out to your sides, feet against the wall.
    Keep your back straight and press your legs into the wall.
2. Reach your arms forward and place your hands on the wall for support.
3. Hold this pose for 20-30 seconds.

Wall Shoulder Stand

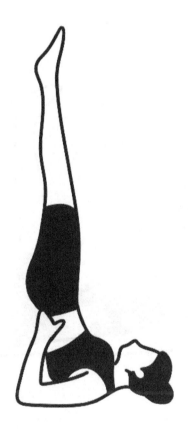

1. Lie on your back and place your feet flat on the wall with your knees bent.
2. Push into the wall to lift your hips off the floor, and place your hands on your lower back for support.
3. Extend your legs upward, pressing your feet into the wall.
4. Hold this position for 30-60 seconds.

Wall Half Happy Baby Pose

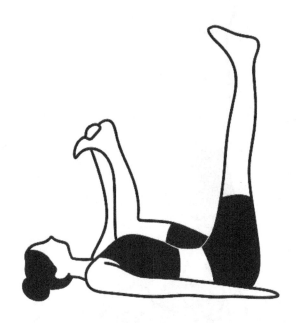

1. Position yourself in a supine posture, lying on your back with your knees flexed and your feet placed flat against the wall.
2. Draw your right knee towards your chest, keeping the left foot on the wall.
3. Hold the outside of your right foot with your right hand. If you can't reach your foot, you can use a strap or belt.
4. Press your right knee towards the wall, opening your hip.
5. Hold this pose for 30-60 seconds, then switch legs.

Half Plough Pose

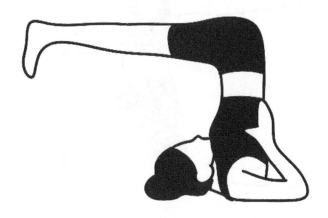

1. Lie on your back and lift your legs up to rest against the wall.
2. Place your hands under your hips for support, and lift them off the floor.
3. Push your legs against the wall as you lift your hips even higher.
4. Try to bring your toes over your head while keeping your legs straight.
5. Hold this pose for 30-60 seconds.

Crescent Low Lunge Pose Twist at Wall

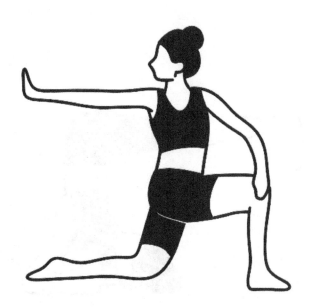

1. Begin the sequence by adopting a low lunge position. Place your right foot forward, bending the knee at a 90-degree angle while allowing your left knee to rest on the floor.
2. Place your hands on the wall, slightly higher than your shoulders.
3. Rotate your upper body towards the right side, simultaneously extending your right arm upward.
4. Look up towards your right hand.
5. Hold this pose for 30-60 seconds, then switch sides.

Revolved Triangle Pose

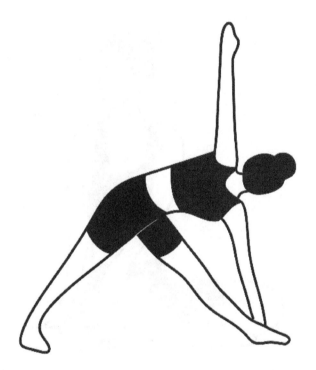

1. Stand a few feet away from the wall, feet hip-width apart.
2. Step your right foot back about three to four feet and place it flat on the floor.
3. Place your left hand on the wall and reach your right arm towards the ceiling, twisting your upper body to the right.
4. Look up towards your right hand.
5. Hold this pose for 30-60 seconds, then switch sides.

Seated Spinal Twist

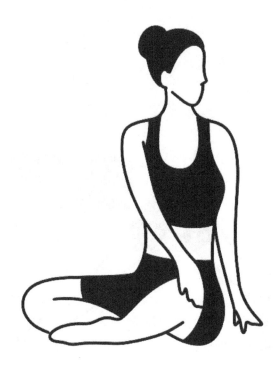

1. Sit with your back against the wall and your legs extended out in front of you.
2. Flex your right knee and cross it over your left leg, positioning your right foot on the ground outside of your left knee. Rotate your upper body towards the right, utilizing your right hand for stability by placing it on the floor behind you while your left arm wraps around your right knee.
3. Press your back into the wall to help deepen the twist.
4. Hold this pose for 30-60 seconds, then switch sides.

Standing Side Bend Pose

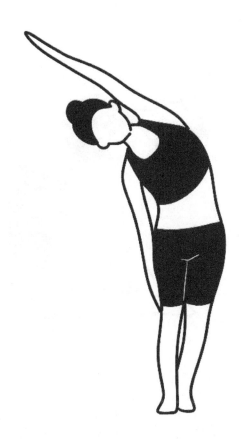

1. Stand with your right side against the wall; feet hip-width apart.
2. Reach your right arm up and place your hand against the wall.
3. Slide your hand up the wall as you bend to your left, stretching the right side of your body.
4. Maintain this posture for a duration of 20 to 30 seconds, then proceed to switch sides and repeat the sequence.

Camel Pose with Strap and Wall

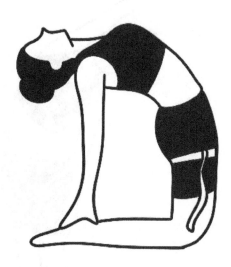

1. Assume an upright posture, facing away from the wall. Secure a yoga strap or belt around your ankles by creating a loop. Lower yourself into a kneeling position, ensuring your knees are positioned at a hip-width distance, and press your feet against the wall.
2. Place your hands on your lower back, fingers pointing down.
3. Begin to lean backward, arching your back and pressing your hips forward.
4. Reach your hands back towards the strap around your ankles. If you can't reach the belt, keep your hands on your lower back.
5. Look straight ahead or gently tilt your head back, depending on your comfort level.
6. Press your feet into the wall for balance and support.
7. Hold this pose for 20-30 seconds. To release, carefully bring your hands back to your lower back and slowly come up.

Garland Pose Back Wall

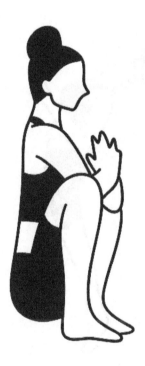

1. Stand with your back against the wall, feet wider than hip-width apart.
2. Gradually flex your knees and descend into a squatting position, ensuring that your back maintains contact with the wall. Press your elbows against the inner sides of your knees and join your palms together at your heart center.
3. Hold this pose for 30-60 seconds.

Cobra Pose

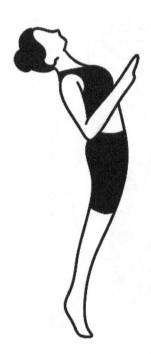

1. Lie on your stomach with your feet against the wall.
2. Place your hands on the floor under your shoulders.
3. Press your hands into the floor and lift your chest, coming into a cobra pose.
4. Press your feet into the wall to deepen the stretch.
5. Hold this pose for 30-60 seconds.

Standing Backbend Pose Hands on Wall

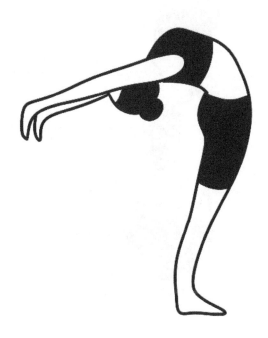

1. Stand a few feet away from the wall, facing away.
2. Reach your arms back and place your hands on the wall behind you.
3. Bend backward, arching your back and pushing your hips forward.
4. Hold this pose for 30-60 seconds.

Seated Wind Release Pose Variation at Wall

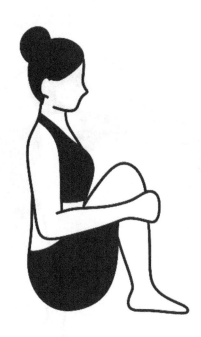

1. Position yourself on the floor, sitting with your legs extended upwards against the wall. Flex your right knee and draw it towards your chest, hugging it in an embracing motion while simultaneously maintaining your left leg extended against the wall.
2. Hold this pose for 30-60 seconds, then switch sides.

Reverse Warrior Pose

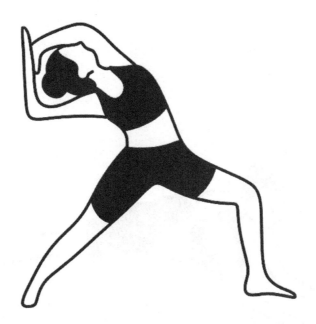

1. Stand in Warrior II with your right knee bent, your left leg straight, and your foot against the wall.
2. Reach your right arm and lean back, placing your left hand on your left leg for support.
3. Hold this pose for 30-60 seconds, then switch sides.

Prone Straddle Split Pose

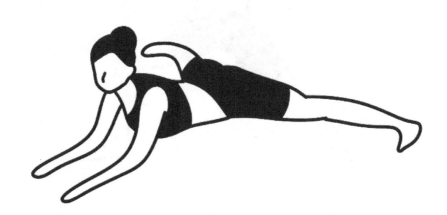

1. Assume a prone position lying on your stomach, and extend your legs upwards against the wall in a wide straddle formation.
2. Relax into this pose and hold for 1-3 minutes.

Supine Hip Hike Feet on Wall

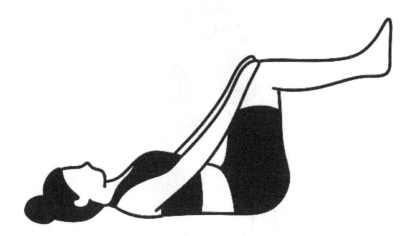

1. Lie on your back with your legs extended up against the wall.
2. Lift your right hip off the floor, then lower it back down.
3. Repeat for 10-15 reps, then switch sides.

Forward Fold Against Wall

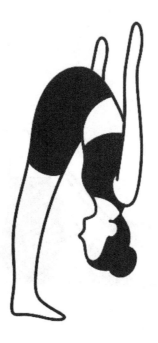

1. Stand facing the wall.
2. Walk your feet back and fold at the hips, reaching your hands to the wall and keeping your legs straight.
3. Relax your head and neck and hold for 30-60 seconds.

Soleus Stretch Pose Against Wall

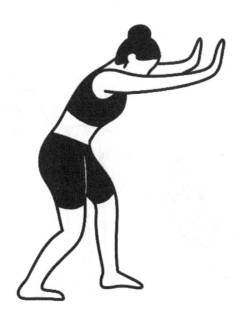

1. Stand facing the wall.
2. Place your right foot back, keeping your heel on the ground and your left foot closer to the wall.
3. Lean into the wall, bending your front knee and keeping your back leg straight.
4. Hold for 30-60 seconds, then switch sides.

One-Legged King Pigeon Pose II

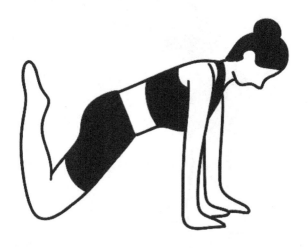

1. Start on your hands and knees, with your back towards the wall.
2. Flex your right knee and bring it forward, positioning it on the ground in proximity to your right hand.
3. Slide your left leg back, resting your left foot and shin against the wall.
4. Fold forward and extend your hands on the floor in front of you.
5. Hold this pose for 30-60 seconds, then switch sides.

Butterfly Pose

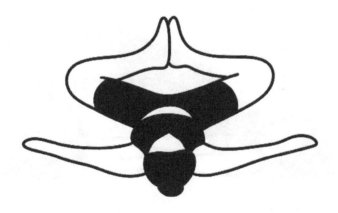

1. Sit down with the soles of your feet together, knees bent out to the sides, and your feet against the wall.
2. Press your knees gently towards the wall using your elbows. Maintain a straight alignment of your spine while simultaneously keeping your shoulders in a relaxed state.
3. Hold this pose for 20-30 seconds.

Bridge Pose Variation Blocks Under Feet

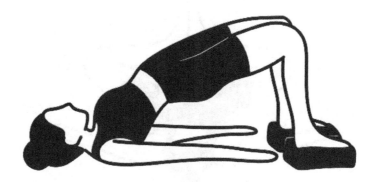

1. Recline on your back, allowing your knees to bend, and position your feet on yoga blocks resting against the wall.
2. Lift your hips off the floor, coming into a bridge pose.
3. Press your feet into the blocks and the wall to lift your hips higher.
4. Hold this pose for 30-60 seconds.

BALANCE EXERCISES

Wall Dead Bug

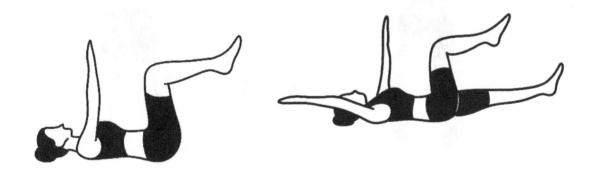

1. Lie on your back and place your feet flat on the wall, knees bent at 90 degrees.
2. Extend your arms up towards the ceiling.
3. Lower your right arm and left leg towards the floor while keeping the other arm and leg in place.
4. Please return them to the initial position and repeat with the other arm and leg.
5. Repeat this Movement 10-12 times (5-6 for each side).

Wall Angels

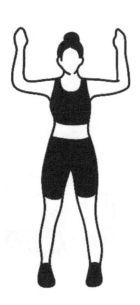 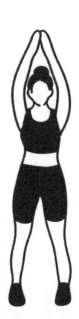

1. Assume a position where your back is in contact with the wall, and your feet are spaced apart at the width of your shoulders.
2. Raise your arms and place them against the wall with your elbows bent at a 90-degree angle, like you're forming the letter 'W'.
3. Slide your arms upwards to form the letter 'I', keeping your wrists and elbows in contact with the wall.
4. Lower them back down to the 'W' position.
5. Repeat this Movement 10-12 times.

Revolved Triangle Pose Against Wall

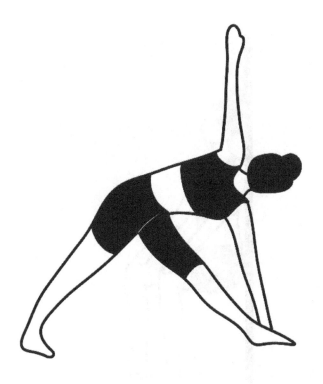

1. Stand a few feet away from the wall, with your back to the wall.
2. Advance your right foot forward and simultaneously move your left foot backward, positioning your left foot against the wall, and exerting pressure on it.
3. Hinge at the hips to fold forward, reaching your right hand to your left ankle and your left hand against the wall.
4. Turn your gaze towards your left hand, hold for 30-60 seconds, then switch sides.

Wide-Legged Chair Pose Back

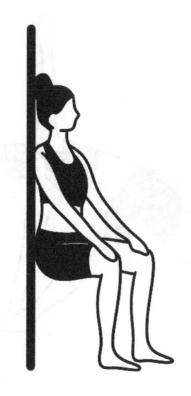

1. Stand with your back against the wall and feet hip-width apart.
2. With a wide stride, move your feet apart and flex your knees, progressively lowering your back along the wall until your thighs reach a parallel position to the floor. Extend your arms forward in a parallel position to the floor.
3. Hold this pose for 30-60 seconds.

Tree Pose Hand

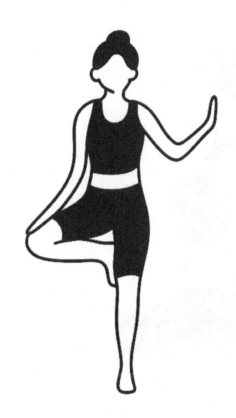

1. Stand a few feet away from the wall, facing it.
2. Transfer your weight onto your right foot and place the sole of your left foot against the inner part of your right thigh. Extend your arms, raise them overhead, and press your palms firmly against the wall.
3. Hold this pose for 30-60 seconds, then switch sides.

Staff Pose Wall

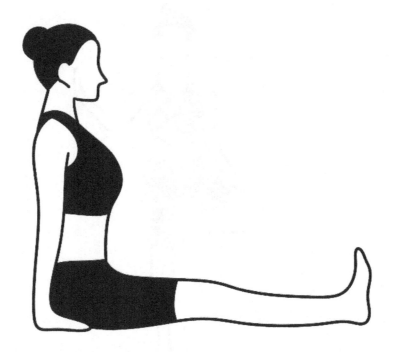

1. Position yourself on the floor, sitting with your legs extended forward and your back resting against the wall. Press your hands firmly into the floor beside your hips and flex your feet, pushing your heels away from your body. Activate your core muscles and press your lower back against the wall to create engagement.
2. Hold this pose for 30-60 seconds.

Standing One Leg Raised Pose Wall Hip Hike

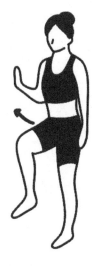 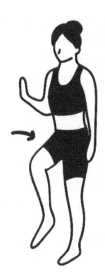

1. Assume a standing position while facing the wall, and position your right foot against the wall, ensuring that your leg remains straight.
2. Slowly lift your left hip as high as possible, then slowly lower it back down.
3. Repeat for 10-15 reps, then switch sides.

BEGINNER'S WEEKLY PROGRAM

This program is designed for beginners, people recovering from injuries, and the elderly. It incorporates a blend of strength, flexibility, balance, and warm-up exercises, ensuring a holistic workout while minimizing strain. Each session should last approximately 10 minutes.

Day 1 - Warm-Up & Strength Focus
1. Wall Mountain Climbers - 60 seconds
2. Wall Lunges - 60 seconds
3. Wall Plank - 60 seconds
4. Wall Push-Ups - 60 seconds
5. Wall Sit With Mini Fitness Ball - 60 seconds
6. Downward Dog - 60 seconds
7. High Lunge Pose - 60 seconds (30 seconds on each side)
8. Wall Tuck and Extend - 60 seconds
9. Wall Dead Bug - 60 seconds
10. Eye of The Needle Pose - 60 seconds (30 seconds on each side)

Day 2 - Flexibility & Balance Focus
1. Wall Downward Facing Dog - 60 seconds
2. Legs Up The Wall Pose - 60 seconds
3. Sleeping Pigeon Pose - 60 seconds (30 seconds on each side)
4. Half Plough Pose - 60 seconds
5. Tree Pose Hand - 60 seconds (30 seconds on each side)
6. Seated Spinal Twist - 60 seconds (30 seconds on each side)
7. Standing Side Bend Pose - 60 seconds (30 seconds on each side)
8. Butterfly Pose - 60 seconds
9. Wall Shoulder Stand - 60 seconds
10. Garland Pose Back Wall - 60 seconds

Day 3 - Rest and Recovery

Day 4 - Strength & Balance Focus
1. Wall Handstand - 60 seconds
2. Supported Warrior III - 60 seconds (30 seconds on each side)
3. Wall Side Plank - 60 seconds (30 seconds on each side)
4. Wall Bridge - 60 seconds
5. Wall Single-Leg Lifts - 60 seconds (30 seconds on each side)
6. Wall Calf Raises - 60 seconds
7. Staff Pose Wall - 60 seconds
8. Wall Sphinx Pose - 60 seconds
9. Wall Angels - 60 seconds
10. Wall Dead Bug - 60 seconds

Day 5 - Flexibility & Warm-Up Focus
1. Wall Leg Swings - 60 seconds (30 seconds on each side)

2. Upward Forward Fold - 60 seconds
3. Wall Slide - 60 seconds
4. Chest Stretch - 60 seconds
5. Straddle Pose - 60 seconds
6. Puppy Dog Pose - 60 seconds
7. Crescent Low Lunge Pose Twist At Wall - 60 seconds (30 seconds on each side)
8. Seated Wind Release Pose Variation At Wall - 60 seconds
9. Standing Backbend Pose Hands On Wall - 60 seconds
10. Soleus Stretch Pose Against Wall - 60 seconds

Day 6 - Rest and Recovery

Day 7 - Mixed Focus (Strength, Balance, Flexibility)
1. Wall Squats - 60 seconds
2. Wall Tuck and Extend - 60 seconds
3. Wide-Legged Chair Pose Back - 60 seconds
4. Cobra Pose - 60 seconds
5. Bridge Pose Variation Blocks Under Feet - 60 seconds
6. Reverse Warrior Pose - 60 seconds (30 seconds on each side)
7. Standing One Leg Raised Pose Wall Hip Hike - 60 seconds (30 seconds on each side)
8. One-Legged Standing Backbend - 60 seconds
9. Forward Fold Against Wall - 60 seconds
10. One-Legged King Pigeon Pose II - 60 seconds

Don't overlook the significance of warming up before your workout and cooling down afterward. Pay attention to the signals your body sends you to avoid overexerting yourself.

CARDIAC HEALTH AND STRESS RELIEF PROGRAM

A healthy heart and a calm mind are key components of overall well-being. This 10-minute program is designed to enhance cardiac health while simultaneously relieving stress. By engaging in gentle physical activity, the heart is strengthened, and the circulation improved. Simultaneously, the concentration and focus needed for these exercises help in reducing stress and promoting mental tranquility.

Before beginning any exercise program, especially if you have heart disease or other health concerns, consult your doctor.

Day 1 - Cardiovascular & Relaxation Focus
1. Wall Mountain Climbers - 60 seconds
2. Wall Push-Ups - 60 seconds
3. Wall Plank - 60 seconds
4. Wall Bridge - 60 seconds
5. High Lunge Pose - 60 seconds (30 seconds on each side)
6. Wall Handstand - 60 seconds
7. Legs Up The Wall Pose - 60 seconds
8. Seated Spinal Twist - 60 seconds (30 seconds on each side)
9. Wall Shoulder Stand - 60 seconds
10. Supine Hip Hike Feet On Wall - 60 seconds

Day 2 - Rest and Recovery

Day 3 - Cardiovascular & Relaxation Focus
1. Wall Squats - 60 seconds
2. Wall Downward Facing Dog - 60 seconds
3. Wall Tuck and Extend - 60 seconds
4. Wall Dead Bug - 60 seconds
5. Wall Side Plank - 60 seconds (30 seconds on each side)
6. Wall Lunges - 60 seconds
7. Tree Pose Hand - 60 seconds (30 seconds on each side)
8. Half Plough Pose - 60 seconds
9. Sleeping Pigeon Pose - 60 seconds (30 seconds on each side)
10. Cobra Pose - 60 seconds

Day 4 - Rest and Recovery

Day 5 - Cardiovascular & Relaxation Focus
1. Wall Mountain Climbers - 60 seconds
2. Wall Single-Leg Lifts - 60 seconds (30 seconds on each side)
3. Wall Bridge - 60 seconds
4. Wall Calf Raises - 60 seconds
5. Supported Warrior III - 60 seconds (30 seconds on each side)
6. Wall Sphinx Pose - 60 seconds
7. Legs Up The Wall Pose - 60 seconds

8. Eye of The Needle Pose - 60 seconds (30 seconds on each side)
9. Standing Backbend Pose Hands On Wall - 60 seconds
10. One-Legged King Pigeon Pose II - 60 seconds

Day 6 - Rest and Recovery

Day 7 - Cardiovascular & Relaxation Focus
1. Wall Push-Ups - 60 seconds
2. Wall Downward Facing Dog - 60 seconds
3. Wall Plank - 60 seconds
4. Wall Dead Bug - 60 seconds
5. Wall Side Plank - 60 seconds (30 seconds on each side)
6. Seated Spinal Twist - 60 seconds (30 seconds on each side)
7. Wall Shoulder Stand - 60 seconds
8. Tree Pose Hand - 60 seconds (30 seconds on each side)
9. Supine Hip Hike Feet On Wall - 60 seconds
10. Cobra Pose - 60 seconds

When required, take intervals of rest, and modify the routine to accommodate your personal abilities and needs better.

PROGRAM TO BOOST FLEXIBILITY

The importance of flexibility as a core aspect of fitness is frequently underestimated. Boosting your flexibility can assist in correcting posture, easing muscle tightness, and lowering the likelihood of injuries.

The following 15-minute program is dedicated to enhancing your flexibility:
Day 1 - Lower Body & Spine Focus
1. Downward Dog - 90 seconds
2. High Lunge Pose - 90 seconds (45 seconds on each side)
3. Legs Up The Wall Pose - 90 seconds
4. Butterfly Pose - 90 seconds
5. Garland Pose Back Wall - 90 seconds
6. Wall Calf Raises - 90 seconds
7. Wall Single-Leg Lifts - 90 seconds (45 seconds on each side)
8. Seated Spinal Twist - 90 seconds (45 seconds on each side)
9. Forward Fold Against Wall - 90 seconds
10. One-Legged King Pigeon Pose II - 90 seconds (45 seconds on each side)

Day 2 - Upper Body & Core Focus
1. Wall Push-Ups - 90 seconds
2. Wall Downward Facing Dog - 90 seconds
3. Wall Plank - 90 seconds
4. Wall Shoulder Stand - 90 seconds
5. Chest Stretch - 90 seconds
6. Wall Angels - 90 seconds
7. Wall Handstand - 90 seconds
8. Wall Sphinx Pose - 90 seconds
9. Standing Backbend Pose Hands On Wall - 90 seconds
10. Cobra Pose - 90 seconds

Day 3 - Full Body Focus
1. Wall Mountain Climbers - 90 seconds
2. Wall Bridge - 90 seconds
3. Wall Tuck and Extend - 90 seconds
4. Wall Dead Bug - 90 seconds
5. Tree Pose Hand - 90 seconds (45 seconds on each side)
6. Standing Side Bend Pose - 90 seconds (45 seconds on each side)
7. Wall Sit With Mini Fitness Ball - 90 seconds
8. Supine Hip Hike Feet On Wall - 90 seconds
9. Staff Pose Wall - 90 seconds
10. Four-Limbed Staff Pose Feet Against Wall - 90 seconds

Day 4 - Hips & Legs Focus
1. Sleeping Pigeon Pose - 90 seconds (45 seconds on each side)
2. Eye of The Needle Pose - 90 seconds (45 seconds on each side)
3. Wall Leg Swings - 90 seconds (45 seconds on each side)

4. Half Plough Pose - 90 seconds
5. Wall Side Plank - 90 seconds (45 seconds on each side)
6. Straddle Pose - 90 seconds
7. Standing One Leg Raised Pose Wall Hip Hike - 90 seconds (45 seconds on each side)
8. Wall Squats - 90 seconds
9. One-Legged Standing Backbend - 90 seconds (45 seconds on each side)
10. Soleus Stretch Pose Against Wall - 90 seconds (45 seconds on each side)

Day 5 - Chest & Shoulders Focus
1. Supported Warrior III - 90 seconds (45 seconds on each side)
2. Wall Slide - 90 seconds
3. Wall Angels - 90 seconds
4. Chest Stretch - 90 seconds
5. Wall Shoulder Stand - 90 seconds
6. Standing Backbend Pose Hands On Wall - 90 seconds
7. Wall Handstand - 90 seconds
8. Wall Sphinx Pose - 90 seconds
9. Wall Downward Facing Dog - 90 seconds
10. Four-Limbed Staff Pose Feet Against Wall - 90 seconds

Day 6 - Spine & Back Focus
1. Bridge Pose Variation Blocks Under Feet - 90 seconds
2. Seated Spinal Twist - 90 seconds (45 seconds on each side)
3. Wall Bridge - 90 seconds
4. Wall Plank - 90 seconds
5. Wall Dead Bug - 90 seconds
6. Wall Sphinx Pose - 90 seconds
7. Wall Handstand - 90 seconds
8. Camel Pose With Strap And Wall - 90 seconds
9. Wall Downward Facing Dog - 90 seconds
10. Cobra Pose - 90 seconds

Day 7 - Relaxation & Recovery
1. Legs Up The Wall Pose - 90 seconds
2. Upward Forward Fold - 90 seconds
3. Butterfly Pose - 90 seconds
4. Seated Wind Release Pose Variation At Wall - 90 seconds
5. Wide-Legged Chair Pose Back - 90 seconds
6. Half Plough Pose - 90 seconds
7. Wall Shoulder Stand - 90 seconds
8. Wall Angels - 90 seconds
9. Puppy Dog Pose - 90 seconds
10. Staff Pose Wall - 90 seconds

These routines help your body recover while still promoting flexibility. The concluding day prioritizes mitigating stress and fostering tranquility, conditioning your body for recovery and the impending week. As you engage in each exercise, remember to take deep breaths, assisting your body to relax and dissipate tension.

BUTT FIRMING AND STOMACH FLATTENING PROGRAM

This 15-minute program focuses on strengthening and toning exercises that target the buttocks and abdomen, helping to firm these areas and improve overall body composition. As always, ensure to consult with a healthcare professional or certified fitness trainer before beginning a new exercise routine.

Day 1 - Core & Glute Focus
1. Wall Mountain Climbers - 90 seconds
2. Wall Plank - 90 seconds
3. Wall Dead Bug - 90 seconds
4. Wall Tuck and Extend - 90 seconds
5. Wall Bridge - 90 seconds
6. Wall Lunges - 90 seconds
7. Wall Single-Leg Lifts - 90 seconds (45 seconds on each side)
8. Wall Sit With Mini Fitness Ball - 90 seconds
9. High Lunge Pose - 90 seconds (45 seconds on each side)
10. Wall Sphinx Pose - 90 seconds

Day 2 - Stretch & Strengthen Focus
1. Wall Downward Facing Dog - 90 seconds
2. Cobra Pose - 90 seconds
3. Half Plough Pose - 90 seconds
4. Seated Spinal Twist - 90 seconds (45 seconds on each side)
5. One-Legged King Pigeon Pose II - 90 seconds (45 seconds on each side)
6. Supported Warrior III - 90 seconds (45 seconds on each side)
7. Standing Backbend Pose Hands On Wall - 90 seconds
8. Forward Fold Against Wall - 90 seconds
9. Bridge Pose Variation Blocks Under Feet - 90 seconds
10. Four-Limbed Staff Pose Feet Against Wall - 90 seconds

Day 3 - Core Activation and Strengthening
1. Wall Plank - 90 seconds
2. Wall Dead Bug - 90 seconds
3. Wall Tuck and Extend - 90 seconds
4. Wall Sit With Mini Fitness Ball - 90 seconds
5. Wall Bridge - 90 seconds
6. Wall Single-Leg Lifts - 90 seconds (45 seconds on each side)
7. Wall Push-Ups - 90 seconds
8. Seated Wind Release Pose Variation At Wall - 90 seconds
9. Wall Sphinx Pose - 90 seconds
10. Wall Mountain Climbers - 90 seconds

Day 4 - Glute Activation and Strengthening
1. Wall Lunges - 90 seconds (45 seconds on each side)
2. Wall Bridge - 90 seconds
3. High Lunge Pose - 90 seconds (45 seconds on each side)

4. Supported Warrior III - 90 seconds (45 seconds on each side)
5. Wall Single-Leg Lifts - 90 seconds (45 seconds on each side)
6. Wall Squats - 90 seconds
7. Standing One Leg Raised Pose Wall Hip Hike - 90 seconds (45 seconds on each side)
8. One-Legged Standing Backbend - 90 seconds (45 seconds on each side)
9. Wall Calf Raises - 90 seconds
10. Wall Downward Facing Dog - 90 seconds

Day 5 - Core & Glute Recovery and Flexibility
1. Downward Dog - 90 seconds
2. Legs Up The Wall Pose - 90 seconds
3. Seated Spinal Twist - 90 seconds (45 seconds on each side)
4. Sleeping Pigeon Pose - 90 seconds (45 seconds on each side)
5. Half Plough Pose - 90 seconds
6. Butterfly Pose - 90 seconds
7. Forward Fold Against Wall - 90 seconds
8. Wall Shoulder Stand - 90 seconds
9. Wall Handstand - 90 seconds
10. Wall Side Plank - 90 seconds

Day 6 - Rest Day
Rest is crucial to recovery and muscle growth. Feel free to engage in gentle stretching or yoga to stay mobile and alleviate muscle stiffness.

Day 7 - Full Body Activation
1. Wall Mountain Climbers - 90 seconds
2. Wall Plank - 90 seconds
3. Wall Tuck and Extend - 90 seconds
4. Wall Bridge - 90 seconds
5. Wall Single-Leg Lifts - 90 seconds (45 seconds on each side)
6. High Lunge Pose - 90 seconds (45 seconds on each side)
7. Wall Dead Bug - 90 seconds
8. Wall Sphinx Pose - 90 seconds
9. Supported Warrior III - 90 seconds (45 seconds on each side)
10. Wall Handstand - 90 seconds

This program blends strength and flexibility training, targeting the muscles in your core and glutes. Remember to engage your core throughout each exercise to maximize the benefits. It's also important to maintain controlled, deep breathing to support your movements and enhance your overall workout experience.

FUN WEIGHT-LOSS PROGRAM

This program is designed to make weight loss fun and engaging! With a blend of strength training, cardio, and yoga exercises, you'll feel energized and motivated. Each session should last approximately 20 minutes. Remember to check with a healthcare professional before starting any new exercise routine.

Day 1 - Cardio Burst & Strength Training
1. Wall Mountain Climbers - 120 seconds
2. Wall Push-Ups - 120 seconds
3. Wall Lunges - 120 seconds (60 seconds on each side)
4. Wall Tuck and Extend - 120 seconds
5. High Lunge Pose - 120 seconds (60 seconds on each side)
6. Wall Handstand - 120 seconds
7. Wall Bridge - 120 seconds
8. Wall Side Plank - 120 seconds (60 seconds on each side)
9. Wall Plank - 120 seconds
10. Wall Dead Bug - 120 seconds

Day 2 - Yoga Flow & Flexibility
1. Downward Dog - 120 seconds
2. Wall Downward Facing Dog - 120 seconds
3. Tree Pose Hand - 120 seconds (60 seconds on each side)
4. Legs Up The Wall Pose - 120 seconds
5. Garland Pose Back Wall - 120 seconds
6. Cobra Pose - 120 seconds
7. Wall Shoulder Stand - 120 seconds
8. Seated Spinal Twist - 120 seconds (60 seconds on each side)
9. Butterfly Pose - 120 seconds
10. Half Plough Pose - 120 seconds

Day 3 - Strength Focus & Cardio Burst
1. Wall Push-Ups - 120 seconds
2. Wall Plank - 120 seconds
3. Wall Mountain Climbers - 120 seconds
4. Wall Bridge - 120 seconds
5. Wall Tuck and Extend - 120 seconds
6. Wall Dead Bug - 120 seconds
7. Wall Side Plank - 120 seconds (60 seconds on each side)
8. Wall Lunges - 120 seconds (60 seconds on each side)
9. High Lunge Pose - 120 seconds (60 seconds on each side)
10. Wall Handstand - 120 seconds

Day 4 - Flexibility & Balance
1. Wall Downward Facing Dog - 120 seconds
2. Legs Up The Wall Pose - 120 seconds
3. Tree Pose Hand - 120 seconds (60 seconds on each side)

4. Half Plough Pose - 120 seconds
5. Standing Side Bend Pose - 120 seconds (60 seconds on each side)
6. Seated Spinal Twist - 120 seconds (60 seconds on each side)
7. Butterfly Pose - 120 seconds
8. Wall Shoulder Stand - 120 seconds
9. Garland Pose Back Wall - 120 seconds
10. Cobra Pose - 120 seconds

Day 5 - Cardio Burst & Strength Training
1. Wall Mountain Climbers - 120 seconds
2. Wall Push-Ups - 120 seconds
3. Wall Lunges - 120 seconds (60 seconds on each side)
4. Wall Tuck and Extend - 120 seconds
5. High Lunge Pose - 120 seconds (60 seconds on each side)
6. Wall Handstand - 120 seconds
7. Wall Bridge - 120 seconds
8. Wall Side Plank - 120 seconds (60 seconds on each side)
9. Wall Plank - 120 seconds
10. Wall Dead Bug - 120 seconds

Day 6 - Yoga Flow & Flexibility
1. Downward Dog - 120 seconds
2. Wall Downward Facing Dog - 120 seconds
3. Tree Pose Hand - 120 seconds (60 seconds on each side)
4. Legs Up The Wall Pose - 120 seconds
5. Garland Pose Back Wall - 120 seconds
6. Cobra Pose - 120 seconds
7. Wall Shoulder Stand - 120 seconds
8. Seated Spinal Twist - 120 seconds (60 seconds on each side)
9. Butterfly Pose - 120 seconds
10. Half Plough Pose - 120 seconds

Day 7 - Rest & Recovery
Take the day off from this program to let your body rest and recover. If you feel like moving, consider a gentle walk or some light stretching. Remember, rest days are crucial for muscle recovery and preventing injuries. Your progress in fitness happens during this recovery period, not just during your workouts! So enjoy this day and be proud of all the hard work you've done during the week.

28-DAY WORKOUT ACCOUNTABILITY AND REFLECTION CHART

Day	Work Completed (Yes/No)	Duration of Workouts	Physical Feelings	Mood
Day 1				
Day 2				
Day 3				
Day 4				
Day 5				
Day 6				
Day 7				
Day 8				
Day 9				
Day 10				
Day 11				
Day 12				
Day 13				
Day 14				
Day 15				
Day 16				
Day 17				
Day 18				
Day 19				
Day 20				
Day 21				
Day 22				
Day 23				
Day 24				
Day 25				
Day 26				
Day 27				
Day 28				

CONCLUSION

Embarking on the journey you've just completed through the pages of this book is the first and often most challenging step towards better health and fitness. The routines and techniques outlined in this comprehensive guide have been carefully designed to help you make the most of an often-overlooked piece of "equipment" - the humble wall. The simplicity, accessibility, and effectiveness of these wall exercises transform ordinary spaces into extraordinary opportunities for personal growth and health improvement.

The variety of exercises compiled in this guide cater to multiple aspects of your fitness journey. They range from strength-building routines to flexibility-enhancing exercises, targeted weight-loss programs, and specialized workouts for toning specific body areas. A variety of workout regimes, meticulously designed to cater to different levels of fitness, provide an opportunity for everyone to enhance their physical health through these potent yet straightforward routines.

A key insight gleaned from this book is the realization that pursuing fitness doesn't necessarily mean dedicating long hours at the gym daily. Instead, it emphasizes the value of consistency. Like drops of water wearing down a stone, consistent and regular exercise, even for a few minutes each day, can yield significant, tangible results over time.

Infusing these workout routines into your everyday schedule - be it right after waking up, during a mid-day break, or before an evening meal - converts these instances into potent catalysts of change. These small but meaningful shifts in our day-to-day routines ultimately drive a large-scale transformation. This realization of the power of consistency forms the cornerstone of your fitness journey.

Moreover, these exercises' inherent simplicity allows you to maintain your routine regardless of where you are or how much time you have. All you need is a sturdy wall and the commitment to better health. Engaging persistently in physical exercise will gradually trigger a transformation in your body, enhancing strength, flexibility, and vitality. In no time, you'll observe a noticeable improvement not only in your physical wellness but also in your mental health, considering the established advantages of frequent workouts in mood elevation and mitigation of stress and anxiety indicators.

I appreciate your dedication and your decision to prioritize a healthier lifestyle. The process of writing this book has been an enriching experience in its own right. Each exercise and program was meticulously chosen and structured, aiming to offer effective, doable routines that can truly impact your life positively. Your voyage through the contents of this book is a reflection of your commitment to fitness and a source of inspiration for others venturing on a similar journey.

In line with this ethos of collective improvement and community, if you find value in this book, kindly consider leaving a favorable review on Amazon. Your input provides not only support for me but also serves as a roadmap for others seeking effective fitness enhancement strategies. Your words can help this simple yet potent method reach others who are seeking a sustainable, accessible way to improve their health.

Equipped with this newfound knowledge, any obstacle you encounter can be converted into a stepping stone toward your fitness objectives. Keep in mind health and happiness constitute a journey rather than a destination, and every small step matters. Here's to a healthier, more robust, and more content you. Let the walls be your guide!

Made in United States
North Haven, CT
13 September 2023

41373286R10050